The 5:2 Diet for Beginners

Using Intermittent Fasting to
Lose Weight and Feel Great Without
Really Trying

DAVID ORTNER

ISBN:150881905X
ISBN-13:9781508819059

To my family

CONTENTS

1. INTRODUCTION

The 5:2 diet is a unique and effective intermittent fasting plan that lets you have your cake and eat it too. Intermittent fasting is a new health and weight loss sensation that, thanks to its incredible success and myriad of health benefits, has skyrocketed in popularity in the last several years. Current research is beginning to shed light on the wide-ranging benefits of intermittent fasting—things like greater metabolic efficiency, improved glycemic control, improved brain function, increased fat burning, increased energy, prevention of life-threatening disease, and increased life span.

The premise behind the 5:2 diet is very simple: participants eat normally for five days and restrict caloric intake to 500 calories (for women) or 600 calories (for men) on the other two, non-consecutive, days. The silver lining of this program, of course, is that you'll have guilt-free freedom in your choice of food for five days of the week, all while enjoying the benefits of a wildly successful diet program. And therein lies the appeal of the 5:2 diet. Rather than limiting calories or restricting foods all of the time, you have the comfort of knowing that, on certain days, you can eat without remorse or paranoia. You therefore feel more optimistic and relaxed and are more likely to stick with the diet.

I am not on a permanent 5:2 schedule, although I know some people who are and who really enjoy it. Instead, I use the program to lose weight quickly when needed and also when my body begins to feel a little sluggish and off-balance. You should do whatever works for you. Before you decide, though, let's take a deeper look at some of the benefits of intermittent fasting, and the 5:2 diet specifically.

It really works. Everyone knows that caloric restriction is one of the main factors of weight loss. When you fast (or cut back drastically on calorie intake), it becomes infinitely easier to reduce your overall caloric intake and, consequently, drop unwanted pounds. In fact, it just sort of happens naturally. Fasting gives your body a chance to lose weight because you're simply eating less.

It simplifies your day. Many of my non-fasting days revolve around food. I spend a couple of hours preparing my meals and snacks for the day and even more time thinking about my hunger, planning when to eat my meals, stopping what I'm doing to eat, and then cleaning up after my meals. Think about all the time you will save on your fasting days, when your preparation, eating, and cleaning time are minimized.

It saves money. Food, especially whole, unprocessed food, is expensive. By cutting your calories back to 25% on your fasting days, you'll be saving not only precious time and energy, but also money.

The weight loss benefits aren't limited to calorie restriction. Fasting promotes stronger insulin sensitivity and increased growth hormone secretion, two key components for weight loss and muscle gain. In this way, intermittent fasting helps you achieve a double whammy for weight loss.

The mental and physical health benefits are amazing. Recent studies on the benefits of intermittent fasting have found incredible results. Research conducted by the University of California indicates that alternate-day fasting decreased blood pressure, reduced oxidative damage to various tissues and DNA, improved insulin sensitivity and glucose uptake, and decreased fat mass in participants. A study conducted by Great Britain's University Hospital of South Manchester demonstrated that weight loss using an intermittent fasting regimen resulted in greater improvements in insulin sensitivity than a traditional, continuous energy diet. According to research conducted by the University of Leuven, exercising in a fasted state accelerates fat loss. Animal research conducted by the Gerontology Research Center found that increasing time between meals can improve brain health. And researchers from the University of Virginia found that intermittent fasting causes our bodies to go into repair mode and fix damaged cells by inhibitng the production of a growth hormone, IGF-1 which, later in life, speeds up the aging process and the onset of age-related diseases.

Research further indicates that fasting may even help improve mood states in adults. People who have participated in an intermittent fasting eating plan have found that they sleep better and have higher energy and concentration during the day and, as a result, a greater sense of overall wellbeing.

There are dozens of reasons for you to jump on the intermittent fasting bandwagon, whether weight loss, better health, or more energy is your goal. Fortunately, not only is the 5:2 diet a very effective program, it's also a very easy, painless one. Read on to learn more.

2. THE SCIENCE OF INTERMITTENT FASTING

The practice of religious fasting has been around since ancient times. It's only recently, however, that fasting for health and weight loss has gained mainstream popularity, and for good reason, given the incredible health and weight loss benefits accompanying the practice. But before you dive into an intermittent fasting program headfirst, it's important to reach a general understanding of how, exactly, intermittent fasting affects your body.

Your body operates differently when you are "feasting" versus when you are "fasting." Every time you eat a meal, your body spends a few hours processing that food, burning what it can from what you just consumed. Because it has access to all of this readily-available energy (i.e. the food you just ate), your body will choose to use that food as energy rather than the fat you have stored. This is especially true if you just consumed carbohydrates (including carbohydrates in the form of sugar), because your body prefers to burn sugar as energy before any other source.

During the "fasted" state, on the other hand, your body is no longer absorbing nutrients from your last meal and instead must rely on its energy stores. Your body has two main sources of energy stores: glycogen stores in the liver, which is broken down into glucose and released into the blood for use, and body fat, which is broken down into free fatty acids to be used as energy by many of your cells. Because, when you fast, your body has little recently-consumed food to use as energy, it is more likely to pull from the fat stored in your body, rather than the glucose in your blood stream or glycogen in your muscles and liver. And burning fat, if weight loss is your objective, is a GOOD thing. Expect double the benefits when you exercise in a fasted state, since your body will be forced to use even more of the only source of energy available to it—the fat stored in your cells.

So why does this work? Well, our bodies react to energy consumption (eating food) with insulin production. Essentially, the more sensitive your body is to insulin, the more likely you'll be to use the food you consume efficiently, which can help lead to weight loss and muscle creation. Very importantly for our purposes, the body is most sensitive to insulin during and following a period of fasting. Your glycogen is depleted during fasting, and will be depleted even further during physical exercise, which can further increase insulin sensitivity. This means that a meal eaten during or immediately following fasting will be stored most efficiently: mostly as glycogen for muscle stores, burned as energy immediately to help with the recovery process, with minimal amounts stored as fat.

In other words, intermittent fasting can help teach your body to use the food it consumes more efficiently. And that, my friends, is a key to permanent weight loss.

3. IS INTERMITTENT FASTING FOR YOU?

Intermittent fasting isn't for everyone. There are people for whom it just won't work. Your specific health needs, exercise and nutritional experience, and lifestyle should determine whether you try the 5:2 diet. If you're new to exercise and nutrition, I strongly recommend that you learn the essentials first. Here are some resources to get you started:

http://www.webmd.com/fitness-exercise/the-abcs-of-weight-loss
http://exercise.about.com/cs/weightloss/a/howtoloseweight.htm
http://www.fitocracy.com/knowledge/weight-loss-101/

No diet or fitness regimen should be torturous, and if you're one of those people who, when fasting, gets so hungry that it affects your ability to function normally, you may be best served by another program. And that's fine. You can and should experiment with other methodologies to achieve your goals. Otherwise, if you're a healthy adult who exercises regularly, whether you should follow an intermittent fasting protocol or not really depends on how you like to eat and which program best fits your lifestyle.

Please note that pregnant and breast-feeding women, as well as diabetics on medication, should seek medical advice before trying intermittent fasting. And this sort of program is not recommended for teenagers and children, who are likely to miss out on crucial nutrients needed for growth and may be at risk of developing unhealthy eating habits. If you have an eating disorder, you should avoid the 5:2 diet and any other intermittent fasting protocol. The same goes for you if you're already very lean or if you have an intense daily physical activity regimen. If you are on any medication, or have any other concerns, please see your doctor before beginning the 5:2 diet.

Of course, I can't say whether the 5:2 diet will work for you. I just know that, as one piece of my overall weight loss and health strategy, it has worked very, very well for me.

4. TIPS FOR SUCCESS

The thing that most worried me when I first began the 5:2 diet, and one of the primary concerns that I've observed in others, is that intermittent fasting will lead to lower energy, focus, and an uncomfortable, shaky, hungry feeling during 500 calorie days. Would-be participants are understandably worried that they will spend the entire fasting day totally miserable because they haven't consumed nearly as much food as usual, and thus will be ineffective at whatever task it is they are working on.

Fortunately, I can promise you that it's not as bad as it sounds. Yes, the initial transition from constant eating to calorie restriction can be a bit of a jolt to the system (more mentally than physically, I say). However, once you get through the transition, your body can quickly adapt and learn to function just as well on your 500 calorie days. Here are some tips to get the most out of your diet.

Start gradually. If you decide to begin the 5:2 diet, don't put too much pressure on yourself in the beginning. Perhaps begin with a 6:1 diet, or cut back to 1000 calories instead of 500. Give yourself the freedom to ease into the diet, and you'll be less intimidated by it and more likely to stick with it in the long run. And once you've begun, allow yourself some flexibility. There will be some 500-calorie days that turn into 1000-calorie days. It happens, sometimes unavoidably. Just do your best.

Focus on the purpose of the diet. Think about the outcome you'd like to achieve, but also think about the process. On fasting days, picture your ideal body and remember that your body is dipping into its fat reserve for energy and repairing damaged cells. Let that knowledge encourage and support you. Feel your food addiction weakening its hold on you.

Expect ups and downs. They happen. You'll have really bad days, where you totally blow your calorie count. There will be a birthday party at work, and you'll have a piece of cake. Or two. Or three. You and your friends will head out for an impromptu happy hour and you'll drink three times your day's calorie limits. Your partner will surprise you by making your favorite dinner. You'll have a bad day and drown your sorrows in a hot fudge sundae. These things are part of life, and part of the process. The occasional slipup will not defeat you. By staying open-minded and not panicking during the "downs" you'll figure out how to have more "ups."

Learn to be comfortable with hunger. Learn the difference between "head hunger" and "body hunger." One is your body sending a signal, the other is a symptom of your psyche and, in many cases, a symptom of an addiction to food. Learn not to fear hunger. Remember that, on fasting days, although you are experiencing hunger, your body is hard at work improving insulin sensitivity and re-calibrating your body's use of stored fuel. If you feel tired, low in energy, irritable and headachy, drink plenty of water and eat small portions of oats, whole grains, or lean protein. On non-fasting days, respect and enjoy the process and the privilege of eating.

What you DO eat is as important as what you DON'T. On non-fasting days, don't worry about counting calories, but be sure to eat good quality, nutrient-rich foods. Don't think of non-fasting days as days during which you can eat literally whatever you want. Instead, view them as ordinary days. Don't eat more than you normally would, otherwise you may have trouble achieving your weight loss goals.

Exercise, but don't overdo it. If weight loss is your primary objective, you'll lose the most weight by combining exercise with the 5:2 diet, even on 500-calorie days. Don't overdo it, though. Avoid very intense or endurance-based activity on these days. Listen to your body and don't give it more than it can handle.

Commit to the diet. While you can and should allow yourself flexibility and time to adjust to the 5:2 diet, if you don't eventually fully commit to following it, you won't see the benefits. If you find yourself consistently (rather than occasionally) breaking the diet, look at your behavior and try to determine what triggers your breakdowns. For example, if you follow the diet all day at work, when you only have access to the food you've brought with you, but you find yourself overeating at home, try to stay busy at home or post incentivizing reminders around your kitchen to dissuade you from grazing. Get rid of the food in your kitchen that triggers overeating or compulsive snacking. Prepare ahead of time low-calorie snacks and meals to make your 500-calorie days as easy and thoughtless as possible.

Hunger will happen, but you can minimize it. When you restrict yourself to 500 calories for a day, you will feel hungry. It's unavoidable. In fact, I submit that hunger is an inevitable part of any effective weight loss program. Thankfully, there are some really great ways to help curtail that hungry feeling.

- Always eat protein and fiber in the same meal. It will help you to feel fuller longer. Some great sources of protein: lean meat, such as poultry or fish, eggs or egg whites, and nonfat Greek yogurt. For fiber, try leafy green vegetables, whole grains, and fruits with edible skins.
- Chew sugar free gum. Scientists have found that chewing gum suppresses the appetite, especially for sweet foods.
- Drink tons of water. Water is great for staving off hunger because it fills your stomach, making you feel full. Tea and coffee (without cream and sugar) are fine as well. If you can't live without diet soda, that's fine too, although I generally advise against it. Avoid fruit juices, which often contain lots of sugar.
- Savor every mouthful. People who watch TV or use their computer or phone when they eat feel less full after eating and get hungry sooner than those who pay full attention to their meal.

One of the main purposes of the 5:2 diet is to build self-discipline for dealing with hunger and breaking food's psychological hold over you. If you cave every time you feel hungry, you'll never achieve your goals, so unless the hunger reaches a point where you feel weakened or shaky, find ways to deal with your hunger. Remember, it's just two days a week. You can do it!

5. FREQUENTLY ASKED QUESTIONS

The 5:2 diet is a relatively significant lifestyle change (although not as severe as many other diets) and should not be undertaken without due consideration and preparation. Here are some common questions posed by people participating in and preparing to participate in the 5:2 diet.

Will My Body Go Into Starvation Mode?

We've all heard about "starvation mode." This is the state our body goes into when deprived of fuel for too long a time, where the body believes it is being starved and drastically reduces its metabolic speed. This is a real phenomenon, obviously, but fortunately, there is no need to worry that your body will even approach starvation mode on the 5:2 diet. Studies indicate that the body's metabolic rate doesn't begin to decline until after 60 hours of pure fasting (not just calorie restriction) have passed, and even then, the reduction was only 8%. True "starvation" in the eyes of the body occurs at about 3 days (72 hours) of not eating at all, at which point the primary source of energy becomes the breakdown of proteins, and muscle specifically.

How Much Weight Will I Lose on the 5:2 Diet?

It seems that, for most people, the weight loss averages out to about a pound a week. Of course, the amount of weight you lose will depend on a number of factors, including the types of foods you eat on your non-fasting days and your activity level.

How Will I Feel When I'm Fasting?

Honestly, the first few weeks may be difficult. But it really does get much easier with each fast you do. You will, of course, feel hungry, but this is natural and it comes in waves. I want to reassure you that the hunger does not get worse and worse. The feeling will pass. When I first began the program, I experienced headaches, irritability, and a little shakiness on my 500 calorie days. It wasn't fun, but it passed, and I no longer experience those symptoms. So relax, drink plenty of water (sometimes, the headaches and shakiness are due to dehydration) and remember the ultimate goals of your diet.

Should The 500-Calorie Days Be Consecutive?

No. In fact, it's recommended that you split the 500-calorie days up (for example, Monday and Thursday) to make it easier to stick with the diet. Choose whichever days fit your schedule that week.

Should The 500 Calories Be Spread Across The Day Or In 1 Meal?

It's totally up to you. I like to split up the calories throughout the day, often with a 100 calorie breakfast, two 50 calorie snacks, a 150 calorie lunch, and a 150 calorie dinner. You may feel more comfortable eating a large breakfast and then eating very little throughout the day, or saving most of your calories for dinner. Experiment with a plan that works for you.

What Should I Eat On My Non-Fast Days?

Eat as you would normally. Don't binge, but eat when you're hungry. Focus on nutrient-rich foods and, obviously, if weight loss is your goal, avoid foods that are high in fat and sugar. You don't want to fall into bad habits that will affect your fasting days.

Should I Count Calories On Non-Fast Days?

There should be no need to count calories except on fast days. One of the best things about the 5:2 diet is the fact that you don't have to be on a diet at all for 5 days a week. Some people do count calories – either for interest or because they are afraid they may over-compensate on non-fasting days. Again, do what works for you.

Can I Exercise On Fasting Days?

Yes. In fact, you should. Exercise on fast days will help burn off your fat stores even faster. However, it is probably unwise to attempt very intense workouts or endurance events. Also, please be careful to stay hydrated.

Can I Increase My Fast Day Calories If I Exercise?

I usually don't. It's easy to rationalize and overestimate the number of calories burned by exercise. It's much simpler to just stick with your 500 calorie allotment. Of course, if your workout leaves you feeling shaky or faint, eat a little something extra.

Can I Fast More Or Less Often?

Sure. If you're looking for faster and greater weight loss, you could move to a 4:3 diet (fasting 3 days per week) or if the 5:2 diet is too hard on you, you could try a 6:1 diet. Do what works for you and your body.

Should I Fast If I Am Ill?

I wouldn't. Some people might tell you differently. I've heard colleagues claim that fasting during illness quickens recovery time. That may be true, but I worry about putting any extra strain on the body when it's fighting an illness. I don't exercise when I'm sick for the same reason.

What About Carbohydrates and Sugar?

I've found that a diet high in carbohydrates and sugar makes fasting MUCH more difficult, with more side effects, such as headaches and feeling shaky. There is also some evidence that a diet high in carbohydrate prevents the body from entering repair mode. I would try to avoid sugar as much as possible and seek out carbohydrates in the form of fruits, oats, and whole grains only.

Reach Out To Me

- Do you have a question or comment for me?
- Would you like to make a suggestion for my next book?
- Would you like to receive free weight loss and fitness tips right to your inbox?
- Want to have exclusive access to my FREE Kindle books?

Then send me an email: thedavidortner@gmail.com
I love to get messages from readers and I do my best to send a timely and thoughtful response!

6. FASTING DAY FAVORITES

Five hundred calories is not a lot of calories to play with, so it's important to make every calorie work on your fasting days. That means choosing nutritionally rich foods that will be filling and satisfying for you. The key here is prioritizing three dietary components for weight loss: water, protein, and fiber. All three of these will fill you up before they fill you out.

Water

Drink a LOT of water on your 500 calorie days (and the other five days, for that matter). Drink a glass when you wake up. Drink a glass when you feel hungry. Drink a glass 15 minutes before your meals and snacks. Drink a glass during your meals and snacks. Drink a glass before you go to bed. Water fills your stomach and diminishes the impact of hunger cravings, plus it's very important to make sure you don't get dehydrated during the 5:2 diet.

I also drink a lot of tea on my fasting days, especially in the morning (coffee is fine too, as long as you add no sugar and no, or minimal, cream). Some of my favorite teas include green tea, white tea, chamomile tea, ginger tea, lemon tea, and peppermint tea. All of these teas, I've found, decrease hunger cravings and detoxify the body.

Sometimes, in the evenings, instead of a cocktail, I'll have a glass of sparking water infused with fruits—strawberries, cucumbers, and citrus fruits are my favorite for this purpose.

Protein

I base my 500 calorie day meals and snacks largely around protein. Protein helps keep you feeling fuller for longer, and, if you choose the right protein sources, can be very low-calorie. One egg, for example, only costs you 75 calories. For even fewer calories and less fat, scramble up some egg whites. A few slices of turkey breast cold cuts? A mere 30 or 40 calories. A three ounce chicken breast? Just over 100 calories. Half a cup of nonfat Greek yogurt will net you well under 100 calories. 15 almonds will cost you around 100 calories for a nutritionally dense and satisfying snack, as will a handful of pistachios.

Fiber

Since it's a good idea to steer clear of grain-based carbohydrates on your fasting days, most of your fiber on these days will come from nutrient-rich fruits and vegetables. Fiber is very important for fasting days because it fills you up and cleans you out. And, fortunately, fruits and especially vegetables are very low calorie. Seven stalks of celery are only 45 calories. One apple is just 75 calories. Twelve strawberries, only 48 calories. A large tomato will net you a mere 33 calories. Watermelon is a delicious, satisfying, sweet treat and 2 cups contain less than 100 calories. Sweet prunes are another one of my favorites. They're very high fiber (hence, their reputation for their ability to get things moving) and 4 prunes are less than 100 calories. Raspberries, blueberries, and blackberries are just a calorie a piece. Cherries and snap peas, just 2 calories a piece. Grapes, strawberries, and cherry tomatoes, only 3 calories per fruit.

Foods To Avoid

As we've discussed, it's best to avoid sugar and carbohydrates on your fasting days. They can do nasty things to your blood sugar, causing you to feel tired and shaky, plus they're often much higher-calorie than other foods. I would also advise restricting your intake of fats or oils on 500 calorie days. Fats and oils are good for you in moderation, but they also usually contain lots of calories. For example, there are an incredible 120 calories in just one tablespoon of olive oil. And that one tablespoon certainly isn't going to cause you to feel full or satisfied. Same thing with butter and other high-fat foods and condiments. You're just not getting the bang for your calorie buck with these oils. Save them for your non-fasting days.

My 5:2 Secret Weapon

Soup is a fasting-day lifesaver for me. It's hot, which makes for a more psychologically satisfying meal than a cold, raw meal. It's liquid-based so it fills the stomach well, and if you use a low fat broth, like chicken or vegetable broth, soup is very low-calorie. A cup of homemade chicken soup is only 86 calories. My favorite vegetable soup is just 90 calories. And healthy, soy-based miso soup clocks in at a mere 35 calories. Bonus points if you enjoy plenty of fiber-rich vegetables with (or in) your soup.

Now that you've got a pretty good idea of the types of food you should gravitate to on your fasting days, it's time to hit the grocery store! Here's a shopping list that should cover everything you need for a successful 5:2 week.

5:2 Shopping List For Success

Flavor Enhancers
• Black pepper
• Garlic
• Ginger
• Chiles
• Fresh herbs
• Your favorite spices

Low-Calorie Fruits
• Raspberries
• Blueberries
• Blackberries
• Strawberries
• Cherries
• Apples
• Grapes
• Plums
• Sweet prunes
• Honeydew melon
• Cantaloupe melon
• Watermelon
• Peaches
• Apricots
• Lemon and limes for flavoring
• Bananas
• Tomatoes
• Cherry tomatoes

Vegetables

- Cucumbers
- Celery
- Snap peas
- Green, red, and yellow peppers
- Carrots
- Asparagus
- Green beans
- Onions
- Mushrooms
- Cabbage
- Lettuce
- Spinach
- Zucchini
- Broccoli

Protein
- Boneless, skinless chicken breasts
- Sliced turkey breast
- Turkey bacon
- Salmon and/or tilapia fillets
- Tuna (I like canned tuna for the convenience)
- Shrimp
- Eggs
- Egg whites
- Almonds
- Pistachios
- Nonfat Greek yogurt
- Nonfat or low-fat cottage cheese
- Nonfat or low-fat mozzarella and cheddar cheese
- Parmesan cheese

Miscellaneous
- Chicken broth or stock
- Vegetable broth or stock
- Miso soup (found in the Asian food section of your grocery store)
- Low-calorie and low-fat canned soups
- Salsa
- Steel-cut oatmeal
- Whole grain pitas
- Red wine vinegar and balsamic vinegar to dress salads
- Other low-calorie salad dressings
- Soy sauce
- Herbal teas

- Skim milk
- Sparkling water

7. FASTING DAY MEAL PLANS

Eating 500 calories a day and feeling satisfied is not as hard as you might think, as long as you're careful to choose the right foods and combinations of foods. These meal plans provide a great mix of fruits and veggies that will keep you feeling full and satiated. Some of the plans provide for a fasting day totaling a little over 500 calories, some a little under. There will never be a day during which you eat exactly 500 calories. The key is to stick as close as possible to the goal. Recipes for those items with asterisks are included in the next chapter.

Week 1, Day 1

Breakfast
½ cup plain, nonfat Greek yogurt (65 calories)
½ cup mixed berries (30 calories)

Snack
*Turkey and Cucumber Roll-Up (70 calories)

Lunch
*Roasted Red Pepper and Tomato Soup (97 calories)
*Green Bean and Mushroom Casserole (83 calories)

Snack
*Cottage Cheese Salad (49 calories)

Dinner
*Zucchini and Egg Bake (40 calories)
1 cup Miso Soup (35 calories)

1 cup raw carrots (50 calories)

Week 1, Day 2

Breakfast
*Banana Smoothie (100 calories)

Snack
*Honeyed Yogurt (100 calories)

Lunch
*Portabella Mushroom Pizza (88 calories)
*Citrus Berry Salad (70 calories)

Snack
*Tuna and Cucumber Slices (40 calories)

Dinner
*Vegetable Soup (32 calories)
*Cheesy Celery Boat (17 calories)
*Melon Salad (24 calories)

Week 2, Day 1

Breakfast
*Oats n' Berries (100 calories)

Snack
*Zucchini Parmesan (52 calories)

Lunch
*Chicken and Vegetable Soup (83 calories)

Snack
½ cup grapes (30 calories)
10 almonds (70 calories)

Dinner
*Chili Lime Shrimp (80 calories)
1 cup steamed mixed vegetables (50 calories)

Week 2, Day 2

Breakfast
2 slices turkey bacon (70 calories)
1 cup watermelon, cubed (46 calories)

Snack
1 cup red, yellow, and green peppers, sliced (40 calories)
½ cup nonfat plain Greek yogurt (65 calories)

Lunch
*Vegetarian Potato Soup (56 calories)
Garden salad dressed with vinegar (no croutons, cheese, or meat) (35 calories)

Snack
10 cherry tomatoes (30 calories)
4 slices turkey breast (45 calories)

Dinner
*Mushroom Omelet (100 calories)
½ cup snap peas, steamed (40 calories)

Week 3, Day 1

Breakfast
½ cup egg whites, scrambled (67 calories)

Snack
*Tuna and Broccoli Salad (144 calories)

Lunch
*Vegetable Stir-Fry (140 calories)

Snack
1 apricot, sliced (17 calories)

Dinner
*Cheesy Tomatoes (100 calories)
1 cup diced tomato, cucumber, red onions, tossed with balsamic vinegar (50 calories)

Week 3, Day 2

Breakfast

½ whole wheat English muffin with 1 tablespoon peanut butter (140 calories)

Snack
*Berry Swirl (70 calories)

Lunch
*Onion, Carrot, and Ginger Soup (50 calories)
Spinach leaves tossed with cherry tomatoes and red wine vinegar (50 calories)

Snack
4 sweet prunes (100 calories)

Dinner
3 ounce grilled chicken breast, boneless and skinless (100 calories)
1 cup steamed broccoli (60 calories)

Week 4, Day 1

Breakfast
*Rainbow Fruit Salad (100 calories)

Snack
*Berry Swirl (70 calories)

Lunch
3 ounce grilled salmon fillet (110 calories)
Steamed vegetables (30 calories)

Snack
1 cup baby carrots (52 calories)
1 tablespoon hummus (25 calories)

Dinner
*Asparagus wrapped in Turkey Bacon (75 calories)
*Creamy Broccoli Soup (80 calories)

Week 4, Day 2

Breakfast
Medium boiled egg with 3 asparagus spears (93 calories)

Snack
*Melon salad (24 calories)

Lunch
*Egg, Spinach, and Tomato Scramble (120 calories)

Snack
*Turkey and Cucumber Roll Up (70 calories)

Dinner
Grilled chicken breast open-faced sandwich (200 calories)
½ cup grapes (30 calories)

8. RECIPES

Please note that many of these recipes make several servings. Obviously, it's important that you stick to the correct serving size if you want to stay within your calorie limits. Enjoy!

Main Dishes

Asparagus Wrapped In Turkey Bacon

75 calories
Makes 1 serving

Ingredients

- 12 asparagus spears
- 2 slices turkey bacon
- Freshly ground black pepper
- 1 lemon wedge, to serve (optional)

Directions

Cook the asparagus in a pan of simmering water for 4 to 5 minutes, depending on thickness. Cut the bacon in half lengthways so you have 4 long strips. Bake the bacon on a foil-lined baking pan in the over at 400 degrees F for 15 to 20 minutes or until done. Remove the asparagus from the water and divide it into groups of three, then wrap the bacon around the stems. Arrange the wrapped asparagus on a plate, season with pepper and serve with a lemon wedge on the side.

Garlic Shrimp

80 calories
Makes 1 serving

Ingredients

- 12 large shrimp, raw and peeled
- 1 crushed garlic clove
- Fresh parsley, chopped

Directions

Toss shrimp with garlic and parsley. Thread onto skewers, spray with oil and grill until shrimp turns pink and is cooked through.

Mushroom Omelet

100 calories
Makes 1 serving

Ingredients

- 1 egg
- 1 tablespoon skim milk
- ¼ cup sliced mushrooms
- Salt and pepper for seasoning

Directions

Spray a nonstick pan with just a touch of oil and sauté the sliced mushrooms. Beat the egg and milk together. Season, then add egg mixture to the pan with the mushrooms and cook until the egg is set. If you don't like mushrooms, substitute in tomatoes, onions, spinach, zucchini, or any other vegetable you enjoy.

Egg, Spinach, And Tomato Scramble

120 calories
Makes 1 serving

Ingredients

- 1 egg
- 1 tablespoon skim milk
- 1 tomato, chopped

- ¼ cup steamed spinach

Directions

Beat the egg with the milk. Season the egg mixture and scramble it. Mix in the tomato and spinach. Enjoy!

Vegetable Stir-Fry

140 calories
Makes 1 serving

Ingredients

- 1 onion, sliced
- Half of a red pepper, sliced
- Half of a yellow pepper, sliced
- ½ cup broccoli
- ¼ cup shredded cabbage
- 1 tablespoon vegetable stock or broth
- Soy sauce
- Sesame seeds

Directions

Spray a nonstick pan with a touch of oil. Stir-fry the onions, peppers, broccoli, cabbage, and vegetable stock until all of the vegetables are cooked through. Add a splash of soy sauce and sprinkle with sesame seeds.

Portabella Mushroom Pizza

88 calories
Makes 1 serving

Ingredients

- 2 large portabella mushroom caps
- ¼ cup diced tomatoes
- ¼ cup diced peppers
- 2 tablespoons shredded fat-free mozzarella cheese

Directions

Wash the mushroom caps and let dry. Spray the mushroom caps and a baking sheet with cooking spray. Place the caps on the baking sheet, open ends up. Cook at 350 degrees F with no toppings. Remove from the oven and layer the tomatoes, vegetables, and cheese on the caps. Bake again at 350 degrees F for 10 to 15 minutes. Let the caps cool before eating.

Zucchini And Egg Bake

40 calories per serving
Makes 6 servings

Ingredients

- ½ cup buttermilk, low fat
- ¾ cup egg whites
- 1 egg
- 1 teaspoon Italian seasoning
- 1 teaspoon garlic pepper
- 1 dash pepper
- 1 dash salt
- ¼ teaspoon hot sauce
- 2 cloves garlic, chopped
- 1 medium onion, chopped
- 2 medium zucchini, grated

Directions

Preheat oven to 350 degrees F. Spray an 8 inch square casserole dish with cooking spray. In a large saucepan sprayed with cooking spray, sauté the zucchini, onion, garlic, and dry seasonings until tender, approximately 8 to 10 minutes. Take off heat and let cool.

In a bowl, combine the egg whites, egg, milk, and hot sauce. Beat well. Add the egg mixture to the vegetables. Mix and pour into the casserole dish. Bake for 35 to 40 minutes until eggs are puffy and set.

Cheesy Breaded Tomatoes

100 calories
Makes 1 serving

Ingredients

- Two roasted plum tomatoes
- 2 tablespoons breadcrumbs

- A sprinkle of Parmesan cheese

Directions

Top the tomatoes with breadcrumbs and cheese and bake at 350 degrees F for 10 minutes.

Chili-Lime Shrimp

80 calories
Makes 1 serving

Ingredients

- 10 large shrimp
- 1 tablespoon lime juice
- ½ teaspoon chili powder

Directions

Boil or grill the shrimp until cooked through. Toss the shrimp with lime juice, then sprinkle with chili powder.

Soups

Vegetable Soup

32 calories per serving
Makes 12 servings

Ingredients

- 6 cups vegetable broth
- 2 cups shredded cabbage
- 2 cups chopped broccoli
- 2 medium carrots, chopped
- 2 cups cauliflower
- 1 stalk celery, diced
- 2 cups swiss chard, chopped
- 1 medium onion, chopped
- 2 small zucchini, diced
- 1 medium red bell pepper, diced
- 2 teaspoons fresh thyme, chopped
- 2 cloves garlic

- 2 tablespoons fresh parsley, chopped
- ½ ounce lemon juice
- ¼ teaspoon black pepper
- ½ teaspoon salt

Directions

Place garlic, vegetables, thyme and broth into a large soup pot. Cover and bring to a boil over high heat; reduce heat to low and simmer, partly covered, about 10 minutes. Stir in parsley (or chives). Season to taste with salt, pepper and lemon juice (optional). Simmer for 30 minutes.

Chicken and Vegetable Soup

83 calories per serving
Makes 12 servings

Ingredients

- 1 teaspoon pepper
- 1 teaspoon sea salt
- 1 tablespoon olive oil
- 3 cups chopped or diced chicken breast
- 8 cups chicken broth
- 1 cup chopped carrots
- 1 ½ cups chopped celery
- 1 cup chopped onion
- 2 tablespoons Italian seasoning

Directions

Salt and pepper the chicken breasts and cook in a greased skillet until browned on the outside and cooked through. Chop the cooked breasts and set aside.

Heat the olive oil in a soup pot and add onions, salt and pepper. Cook for 3 minutes. Add carrots, celery and Italian seasoning and cook until vegetables start to soften. Add the chopped chicken and chicken broth to the soup pot. Bring to a boil, reduce heat, and cook on low for 1 hour.

Vegetarian Potato Soup

56 calories per serving

Makes 10 servings

Ingredients

- 1 (16 ounce) bag frozen hash browns
- 1 cup chopped onion
- 1 (14 ounce) can vegetable broth
- 3 cups water (or less for thicker soup)
- 1 (10 3/4 ounce) can of each, undiluted
o Cream of celery soup
o Cream of potato soup
  - 2 cups milk
  - 1/4 cup shredded cheddar cheese
  - Salt & pepper to taste

Directions

Combine frozen hash browns, onion, vegetable broth and water in a Dutch oven and simmer for 30 minutes. Stir in cream of celery and cream of potato soups, milk, salt and pepper. Heat until simmering and serve.

Onion, Carrot, and Ginger Soup

50 calories per serving
Makes 8 servings

Ingredients

- 8 cups chicken stock
- 2 cups chopped carrots
- 2 teaspoons ginger
- 2 cups chopped onion

Directions

Slice the onions, peel the carrots, and dice the ginger. Place in a large soup pot, add the chicken stock, and season to taste. Cook on medium-high heat until the carrots are soft (30 to 40 minutes). Puree in a blender and enjoy.

Creamy Broccoli Soup

80 calories per serving
Makes 8 servings

Ingredients

- 1 teaspoon black pepper
- ¼ teaspoon salt
- 1 tablespoon extra virgin olive oil
- 4 cups vegetable broth
- 1 cup water
- ¼ cup lemon juice
- 2 pounds of broccoli, chopped
- 2 cloves garlic, minced
- 1 large onion, finely chopped

Directions

Heat the oil over medium heat in a large nonstick saucepan. Add onion and garlic, reduce heat to low, and cook until softened, about 7 minutes. Add broccoli, salt, and a pinch of pepper. Stir well to coat. Add broth, water, and lemon juice. Increase heat and bring to a simmer. Partially cover, reduce heat to low, and simmer gently until broccoli is very tender, about 25 minutes.

Transfer soup to a blender and puree, in batches if necessary, or use a hand blender. Serve hot, garnished with a small broccoli floret, if desired.

Roasted Red Pepper and Tomato Soup

97 calories
Makes 12 servings

Ingredients

- 2 cups diced tomatoes
- 3 cups tomato sauce
- 2 red bell peppers, diced
- 1 cup celery, diced
- 1 red onion, diced
- 2 carrots, diced
- 2 cups skim milk
- 2 cups water
- 4 cups vegetable broth
- 2 tablespoons olive oil

- 3 gloves garlic, crushed
- Seasonings to taste

Directions

Roast red peppers under broiler, turning often, until skins are blackened and interiors start to soften. Take out and put into a paper bag, sealing them, and allow them to rest at least half an hour before peeling. Skins should slip right off.

Peel and chop onions and celery. Brown onions in a large soup kettle. Add celery, carrots and garlic, along with the broth. Simmer until tender.

Peel peppers and remove seeds. Put into a blender. Add small amounts of cooked veggies from the broth with roasted peppers into the blender, using a bit more broth to liquify them. Return them to the pan. Heat to simmer.

Add remaining water and simmer gently, stirring often. Stir in milk and continue to heat for 20 more minutes. Enjoy!

Sides and Salads

Cottage Cheese Salad

49 calories
Makes 1 serving

Ingredients

- ½ cup low-fat cottage cheese
- ½ tablespoon chopped chives
- 1 celery stalk, chopped

Directions

Combine all of the ingredients in a small bowl and enjoy!

Sesame Green Beans

38 calories
4 servings

Ingredients

- 1 pound fresh green beans, trimmed

- 1 teaspoon salt
- 1 tablespoon soy sauce
- ½ teaspoon ground ginger
- 2 teaspoons olive oil
- 1 ½ teaspoon sesame seeds
- 1 tablespoon rice wine vinegar

Directions

Steam green beans for 10 minutes. When the beans are cooked through but still crisp, place in a serving bowl. Toss the beans with all of the other ingredients and serve.

Tuna & Broccoli Salad

144 calories per serving
Makes 4 servings

Ingredients

- ½ cup broccoli, steamed
- 1 can solid light tuna
- ¼ cup chopped red onion
- 3 tablespoons chopped fresh parsley
- Juice and finely grated zest of 1 lemon
- 1 clove garlic, minced
- ½ tablespoon olive oil
- Salt and pepper to taste

Directions

Drain the tuna and flake. Whisk the oil, lemon juice, garlic, salt and pepper in a medium bowl. Add broccoli, tuna, onion, lemon juice and zest, and parsley. Toss to coat well.

Zucchini Parmesan

52 calories
Makes 1 serving

Ingredients

- 1 cup sliced zucchini
- 1 tablespoon shredded Parmesan cheese

- Butter spray

Directions

Line a cookie sheet with aluminum foil, then coat with some cooking spray. Place the zucchini slices on the pan, then spritz them with the butter spray. Sprinkle on the Parmesan cheese. Broil for a few minutes until the cheese starts to brown.

Green Bean and Mushroom Casserole

83 calories
Makes 8 servings

Ingredients

- 6 cups green beans
- 2 cups fresh mushrooms, diced
- 1 can reduced fat condensed cream of mushroom soup
- ½ cup skim milk
- 2 cloves garlic, crushed
- ½ cup french fried onions.
- Black pepper to taste

Directions

Preheat oven to 375 degrees F. Cut green beans into 1 inch lengths. In a baking dish, combine soup, milk, garlic, and pepper until smooth. Add green beans and mushrooms, stir until coated and evenly distributed. Sprinkle onions on top in an even layer. Bake 30 to 35 minutes, until onions are crispy and sauce is bubbly.

Sweets and Snacks

Melon Salad

24 calories
Makes 1 serving

Ingredients

- ½ cup cubed honeydew melon
- ½ cup cubed cantaloupe melon
- 1 teaspoon ground cinnamon

Directions

Sprinkle honeydew and cantaloupe with ground cinnamon and enjoy.

Cheesy Celery Boat

17 calories
Makes 1 serving

Ingredients

- 1 celery stalk
- 2 tablespoons low-fat cream cheese

Directions

Spread the cream cheese on the celery and enjoy.

Turkey And Cucumber Roll Up

70 calories
Makes 1 serving

Ingredients

- 1 thick slice of turkey breast (or 2-3 thin slices)
- 1 tablespoon nonfat or low-fat cream cheese
- 5 very thin cucumber slices

Directions

Spread the cream cheese on the turkey slices. Add the cucumber slices. Roll up to eat.

Berry Swirl

70 calories
Makes 1 serving

Ingredients

- ½ cup mixed berries
- ¼ cup nonfat plain Greek yogurt

Directions

Stir together berries and yogurt and enjoy.

Rainbow Fruit Salad

100 calories
Makes 1 serving

Ingredients

- ¼ cup blackberries
- ¼ cup raspberries
- ¼ cup cantaloupe chunks
- ¼ cup grapes

Directions

Combine all of the fruits and let sit for 20 minutes before eating.

Salsa-Filled Pita

118 calories
Makes 1 serving

Ingredients

- 2 diced tomatoes
- ¼ cup diced onion
- Crushed garlic
- Chopped parsley
- 1 teaspoon balsamic vinegar
- 1 mini whole wheat pita

Directions

Mix the vegetables, herbs, and vinegar and serve in the pita.

Banana Smoothie

100 calories
Makes 1 serving

Ingredients

- ½ cup sliced banana
- ¼ cup nonfat yogurt
- ½ cup fresh spinach
- Handful of ice

Directions

Blend all ingredients until smooth and enjoy.

Honeyed Yogurt

100 calories
Make 1 serving

Ingredients

- ½ cup nonfat Greek yogurt
- 1 teaspoon honey
- Dash of cinnamon

Directions

Top the yogurt with the honey and cinnamon and enjoy.

Oats n' Berries

100 calories
Makes 1 serving

Ingredients

- 1/3 cup rolled oats
- ¼ cup fresh berries
- Dash of cinnamon

Directions

Cook the oats with water, then top with berries and cinnamon.

Citrus Berry Salad

70 calories
Makes 1 serving

Ingredients

- 1 cup mixed berries (raspberries, strawberries, blueberries, blackberries)
- 1 tablespoon orange or lemon juice

Directions

Toss the berries with the juice and enjoy.

Tuna Cucumber Slices

40 calories per serving
Makes 2 servings

Ingredients

- 1 large cucumber, peeled
- 1 can water-packed tuna
- 2 carrots, diced thinly
- 1 tablespoon light mayonnaise

Directions

Slice cucumber crosswise into 1 inch thick rounds. Mix tuna, carrots and mayo and top the cucumber slices with this mixture. Sprinkle thinly diced carrots over the top. Chill before eating.

9. CONCLUSION

I hope the advice, recipes, and meal plans I've provided in this book will guide you toward a healthier, happier, and slimmer life! Remember, intermittent fasting programs like the 5:2 diet are amazing tools to achieve all sorts of health benefits and weight loss, but intermittent fasting alone is not itself an all-in-one solution for fat loss. Instead, it's a great tool in your toolbox. You'll be happiest with your results when you combine intermittent fasting with a healthy diet of whole, real, nutrient-rich foods and consistent exercise. (While we're at it, I'd also recommend adding in meditation and/or yoga and at least eight hours of sleep per night.)

I encourage you to continue to self-experiment and gradually develop a health strategy that works for you, your goals, and your lifestyle. The 5:2 diet is a great place to start and, for my money, the best bang for your buck as far as weight loss plans go.

I wish you luck in your journey!

ABOUT DAVID

David, a California-based personal trainer and weight loss expert, was once sixty pounds overweight and so out of shape that he could barely climb the flight of stairs to his apartment. After revamping his diet and his approach to physical activity, he is happier, healthier, and eager to help others achieve the same goals. He views physical fitness holistically and is the author of a number of articles, books, and presentations focused on losing weight and developing a healthy, happy lifestyle. In his free time, he enjoys hiking with his wife, playing basketball with his two sons, watching classic 1980's films, and whipping up tasty meals in the kitchen.

25322463R00028

Printed in Great Britain
by Amazon